Read a Bit! Talk a Bit! Cat

Written by Gunilla Denton Cook

Published by Denton Cook Pty Ltd
Copyright Denton Cook Pty Ltd 2013
ABN 5403936874
Sydney Australia
Phone +61 2 9651 3558
Fax   +61 2 9651 3007
Email: dentoncook@bigpond.com
Cover photo by Ced Bradbury

Read a Bit! Talk a Bit! is a series of reading activity books intended for people with dementia and/or Alzheimer's disease. The books start with a short article for the group to read, followed by a number of questions for the group leader to ask and engage the participants in conversation to encourage personal and meaningful reminiscences to flow.

All the reading pages are in large type, 44 pt, and the text is only on one page per spread in order to help the individual to concentrate on the text and to minimise the constraints of visual impairment.

Memories recalled from earlier in life are often very therapeutic for all and especially for people with memory impairment. These questions are formulated to create meaningful engagement with the past. Remembering increases self esteem and a feeling of positive worth as the participants recall personal experiences.

This series of books successfully achieve this thanks to the range of familiar topics and questions to prompt and encourage discussions.

Titles available:

At the Movies	**Lawnmower**	**Scissors**
Cake	**Money**	**Soup**
Cat	**Pencil**	**Stamps**
Chickens	**Perfume**	**Teddy Bear**
Dog	**Safety Pin**	**Telephone**
Garden	**Sandwich**	

Cats have found their way into most civilisations around the world and continue to be loved by their owners.

Pass to next reader

Read a Bit! Talk a Bit! Cat written by Gunilla Denton Cook.
©2013 Denton Cook Pty Ltd

Cats are often considered to be useful to keep vermin at bay, but these days most cat owners keep them as companions.

Pass to next reader

Read a Bit! Talk a Bit! Cat written by Gunilla Denton Cook.
©2013 Denton Cook Pty Ltd

Domesticated cats have been adored by different cultures for thousands of years. The Egyptians are known to have been cat lovers from paintings that still exist today.

Pass to next reader

Read a Bit! Talk a Bit! Cat written by Gunilla Denton Cook.
©2013 Denton Cook Pty Ltd

It is generally thought that the Romans introduced the domesticated cat to Europe in the first century. This may not be the case.

Read a Bit! Talk a Bit! Cat written by Gunilla Denton Cook.
©2013 Denton Cook Pty Ltd

There is a different school of thought that tells us that cats were already in Europe in the Iron Age, three thousand years ago.

**Pass to next reader**

In 2004 a grave was discovered on Cyprus that contained the skeletons of a man and a cat together. That find is considered to be more than nine thousand years old.

Pass to next reader

Read a Bit! Talk a Bit! Cat written by Gunilla Denton Cook.
©2013 Denton Cook Pty Ltd

16

Cats are found in mythology and there are many superstitions around them. We have all heard that a black cat crossing our path means bad luck.

Pass to next reader

In most western countries cats are said to have nine lives, but there are some European countries that believe they only have seven lives.

Pass to next reader

Read a Bit! Talk a Bit! Cat written by Gunilla Denton Cook.
©2013 Denton Cook Pty Ltd

20

Today cats come in many varieties. They have been bred to our preferences. There are many different furry breeds with long and short hair.

Pass to next reader

Read a Bit! Talk a Bit! Cat written by Gunilla Denton Cook.
©2013 Denton Cook Pty Ltd

There is even a hairless cat for those who love cats, but are allergic to their fur.

Domestic cats come in different sizes, and different colours.

Pass to next reader

Read a Bit! Talk a Bit! Cat written by Gunilla Denton Cook.
©2013 Denton Cook Pty Ltd

There is enough variety for all to find their perfect cat. There are more than five hundred million cats in the world today to choose from.

**Pass to group leader**

Questions

1. How many cats did you have when you were a child?

2. What colour was your favourite cat?

3. What was your cat's name?

4. How often did you try to brush it? Did it like being groomed?

5. What did you feed the cat?

6. Where did your cat sleep?

7. Did your cat ever get into trouble? If so, what did it do?

8. Can you think of a cat's name for every letter in the alphabet?

   A. Angel
   B. Bella, Blacky
   C. Charlie, Chloe, Coco
   D. Daisy
   E.
   F. Felix
   G. Ginger
   H. Harry
   I. Inky
   J. Jasper
   K. Kitty
   L. Lily, Lucy

Read a Bit! Talk a Bit! Cat written by Gunilla Denton Cook.
©2013 Denton Cook Pty Ltd

M. Max, Millie, Milo, Missy, Misty, Molly
N.
O. Oscar
P. Poppy, Puss
Q. Queeny
R.
S. Sam, Simba, Smokey, Smudge
T. Tiger, Tigger
U.
V.
W.
X.
Y.
Z. Zorro

9.   How many kittens have you taken care of over the years?

10.   What is your trick to get rid of cat hairs on clothes and furniture?

11.   What did your cat do to let you know that it was hungry?

12.   Who fed the cat in your house?

13.   Did your cat ever find any mice to chase? If so, did it bring its prey home?

14.   Did your cat wear a collar? If so, what colour was it? Did it have a bell to warn the birds?

15.   What does it mean when a white cat crosses your path?

16.   How many lives do you think your cat used up?

17.   What kind of personality did your cat have?

18.   What was your cat's favorite toy?

19.   Did your cat have any bad habits?

20.   Did your cat have a particular hiding place?